THE MEDICAL EMPOWERMENT INSTITUTE
PRESENTS
TOP 5 STRATEGIES TO INCREASE CLIENT ENGAGEMENT
LYNN PIERRE JONES JR, PT

MED POWER

Top 5 Strategies to Increase Client Engagement:

How to Empower Clients Help Themselves

Lynn Pierre Jones, JR. P.T.

The Top 5 Strategies to Increase Client Engagement:

How to Empower Clients to Help Themselves

Copyright © 2018 The Medical Empowerment Institute Publications

All Rights Reserved

ISBN 978-1717022448

All rights reserved. No part of this book may be reproduced or transmitted in any form or by any means, electronic, or mechanical, including photocopying or recording, or by an information storage and retrieval system, without permission in writing by the author.

Translations of this work must be approved in writing by the author. Please contact the Medical Empowerment Institute for permission to translate in distribution agreements.

To order more copies for you or your team, go to MedProInstitute.com or contact The Medical Empowerment Institute at (704) 961-9730

First Edition

Top 5 Strategies to Increase Client Engagement:

How to Empower Clients Help Themselves

Lynn Pierre Jones, JR. P.T.

TABLE OF CONTENTS

Preface..8

Introduction..10

Chapter 1: Give To Them First..12

Chapter 2: Illuminate What You Have in Common.......................16

Chapter 3: Make Their Goal Your Priority..................................20

Chapter 4: Use Your Imagination...22

Chapter 5: Expect The Results You Want...................................26

References..30

Recommended Reading..31

About..32

PREFACE

I was inspired to write this book as I was working along side my most recent pair physical therapy students from Wingate University, Courtney Reginald and Brittani Young. What I realized was, they were not trained as to how to influence or encourage clients to engage in their desired activities. In short, when they went to request a person to attend to therapy; all they knew how to do was to walk in the room, introduce themselves, and ask. In some cases that will work but in a lot of cases it does not. When people are hurting, upset, in a strange place, or tired, there is a high likelihood that you will get a lot of refusals. My desire was to train my students to communicate in such a way that it reduces the likelihood of their clients refusing to attend physical therapy sessions. My goal was to add to their tool belt. To give them a number of phrases and a greater number of ways of acting that will increase their chances of getting what they wanted. What I knew was that if they get more patience to do what they wanted them to do, then the patients would get stronger, and intern return to their prior level of function in a shorter timeframe.

I could tell that my students wanted to get a yes every time they went to go get a client, but that just wasn't the case. I observed that once they got a no from the client, there was a pause and somewhat awkward silence. This told me that they had no idea what to say or what to do in order to move the client to a yes. They knew that it was in the clients best interest to participate, but they just didn't know how to communicate that fact.

Sometimes it's not just about getting the client to understand that you are here to help them. Sometimes it is more about the fact of getting the client to like and or trust you at the present moment. When the client sees you approach or when the client comes into your office, they are thinking and running various thoughts throughout their minds. They are thinking, do they feel like enduring whatever it is they think you may have in store for them. For the most part they are not thinking two weeks, or three months, or two years down the line. They are not thinking about the long term affects of them not participating or the long-term benefits of them deciding to participate. Most clients are thinking about what do they feel is best for them right now. And as know, our feelings have a tendency to steer us the wrong way.

Our feelings are designed to direct us to the path of least resistance. They are designed to direct us into the path that provides us with a certain degree a pleasure at the current moment. The issue with this is, no one ever achieved anything great while remaining comfortable.

After about a few weeks of observing my students and attempting to figure out a way to help; I decided to write this book. I wanted to give beginner and seasoned medical professionals additional strategies that they could use to earn the trust, respect and enthusiasm of their clients. I want medical professionals to have the ability to inspire enthusiasm with each and every interaction with their clients. I want clients to feel a pull towards their clinicians, not a feeling that they are being pushed around.

My desire is that you enjoy this book's short simplicity. Please understand I am not attempting to win any awards or to be on any bestsellers list. My goal is simply to give you some of the skills that I have learned, so that you can do, what you do, at a higher level. With that being said let's get started!

Live at Your Best

Lynn Pierre

INTRODUCTION

In The Top 5 Strategies to Increase Client Engagement: How to Empower Clients Help Themselves, I want to simplify the process of increasing client engagement. This is not a game or something that is out of your reach. I believe you can double the engagement you experience with your clients with just these five simple strategies. I believe with 100% certainty that anyone that is a part of the human race can do what I'm asking you to do in this book. To tell you the truth, I believe it is your responsibility. If it is in your power to help someone, I believe you should help them. There are people that have been placed in our care that are suffering. Part of the reason why we selected this profession, I hope, is to stop someone's suffering.

One of my daughters a few years ago had an extremely loose tooth in her mouth. It was bothering her when she ate and she didn't want to pull it out at first. She also didn't want me to touch it. As someone who knew what was best for her, it was my responsibility to sell her on the idea that I should pull out her tooth. I communicated with her that it hurts now, is going to hurt when I pull it, but in the near future it will feel better. In addition to that she would be better because of the process. I am of course and authority figure over my child, as her parent. You are not going to be any of your clients parents, but you are and authority figure over them. You are an expert in this space. They view you as an expert. That is why they have stepped into your facility or into your department. It is now time for you to act as if you know exactly what you're doing and you know what is best for your client. What is best is that they agree to doing whatever it is you are requesting of them. That being said, it is your responsibility to use whatever tools you have to encourage them to agree with your request. If you fail to do all that you can to convince them of the importance of walking in agreement with you, you have failed your responsibility as a clinician. Pay close attention to what I said. I did not say that you failed if they don't agree with you. I said you fail if you don't do everything in your power to convince them to participate with you.

It is time right now for you as a professional to make a commitment to yourself. The commitment is that you will do whatever it takes to end the suffering of your client. As much as it depends on you, you will encourage them using all the tools that you have, to participate with you in providing the most excellent service possible. You will commit to demanding more of yourself in this area. We are not taught how to sell our services to ourselves or to our clients. We also don't take classes on influence. I wrote this short book just to help. There are thousands of books out there that you can read on this very subject and I encourage you to do so. All I ask is that this book is a starting point to your educational journey. I cannot guarantee that you will do as well as I do or as well as any other clinicians. But, I will guarantee that you will do better. This is not about competing with another clinician or competing with your client. This is about competing with yourself. How skilled can you become as it relates to increasing the engagement of your clients? Seek out some of the most difficult clients. The ones that always refuse or give clinicians a hard time. Use some of these tools and strategies with them and be mesmerized by the results. I have demonstrated and taught these skills to many of my students with excellent results. My desire is that you also will have excellent results. Please don't hesitate to email me any questions and any praise reports.

So, without any additional introduction. I present to you the next level of client engagement. Have fun and challenge yourself to improve every single day!!!

Chapter 1

GIVE TO THEM FIRST

Is it a typical day working with clients. The sun is shining and the birds are singing. The high today is 73° and the low is 48°. Knock knock knock, good morning it's me Lynn Jones your physical therapist. It's time to start your physical therapy appointment. I see that you are awake, have finished your breakfast, and you are dressed. Are you ready?

"Well, yes, I would be but..."

Now, whatever comes after this but, are the objections and the hindrances that they see as the reasons to why they will not come with me.

"I just ate and now I need my food to settle. What are we going to do today? I didn't sleep well last night. I just don't feel well. Do you mind if I take the day off? Give me just a few more minutes. If you were me, wouldn't you want to rest a little bit longer? I'm too tired."

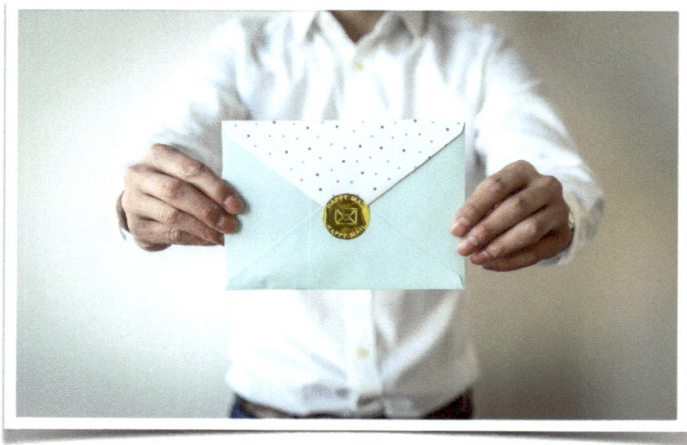

"We must give more in order to get more. It is the generous giving of ourselves that produces the generous harvest." —Orison Swett Marden

The goal here, as you see by the title of the chapter is to give first. What I'm asking you to do here is to remove yourself for a second, from the responsibility of performing your everyday daily task. I know that you are on staff or have the purpose of providing some type of care to your clients. I am not suggesting to you that your responsibilities are not important. What I am suggesting to you is that, if you would like to have another level of compliance, another level of energy, another level of enthusiasm, about your service, there may be a better way. The better way that I am suggesting to you is to prioritize giving something to your client before you make a request of them.

When I speak of giving I am not talking about a physical gift or it could be. I am speaking of giving of yourself. I am speaking of starting a conversation unrelated to the task at hand, just to let them know that you are interested in them as a person. Yes, I want you to perform your exercises, but I also want you to know how your client is doing today and how their evening was last night. By spending a couple of minutes discussing the things that are on the for front of your client's mind. Your client will get the impression, which is true, that you are interested in more than just getting your job done. Giving first positions you to operate at a higher level. A position designed to attract a harvest of compliance from your client. Instead of having to pull teeth and to beg and attempt to manipulate your client into allowing you to provide a service. They will willingly be drawn to whatever it is you're asking them to do.

Based on a conversation with your client you may find out that they have a favorite candy or maybe a favor movie. How much effort would it take for you to bring them that candy or even ask them questions about that movie, so that you could learn more about why it is one of their favorite films. This is not an activity that goes in your daily notes or goes on your task for today. I am challenging you to become an above average clinician by doing the things that the average clinician will not do. I'm asking and requesting you to find pleasure in giving of yourself a little more to your clients.

One day I walked into a clients room with the purpose of giving first. After I knocked and introduced myself, I approached the client who was lying in the bed. I saw that she was already dressed and somewhat appeared to be ready for her therapy appointment. Instead of my first question being "are you ready to get up" or my first statement of "let's get out of bed so you can come to therapy;" I decided to start by asking a question. My question to her was, "is there anything that I can do for you and how are you doing?" As I read her face, which may have been in disbelief, she began to talk about how she wanted to wash her hands in her face. I agreed with her and told her "great let's get that done." I immediately left the room and went to find another coworker that specializes in providing activities of daily living care. My coworker came into the room and not only helped her to wash her hands and her face, but also assessed her ability to wash her hands and her face. So in general this was a win for the patient and a win for my coworker who was able to make and additional assessment of the patient's functional status.

> *"For it is in giving that we receive."* —St. Francis of Assisi

We require and most of the time we request a great deal of compliance from our clients. What I'm saying to you today is that, if your desire is to receive then you must give. Jim Rohn once said that the process of receiving begins with giving. In conclusion, I want you to see if you are thinking from always receiving to prioritizing giving. The next time you have to go and greet a patient or request that a patient performs an activity. Start with giving them something first, It maybe tangible, it may be giving of your time, but give first. Because, it is by you giving that you will receive your harvest.

Chapter 2

ILLUMINATE WHAT YOU HAVE IN COMMON

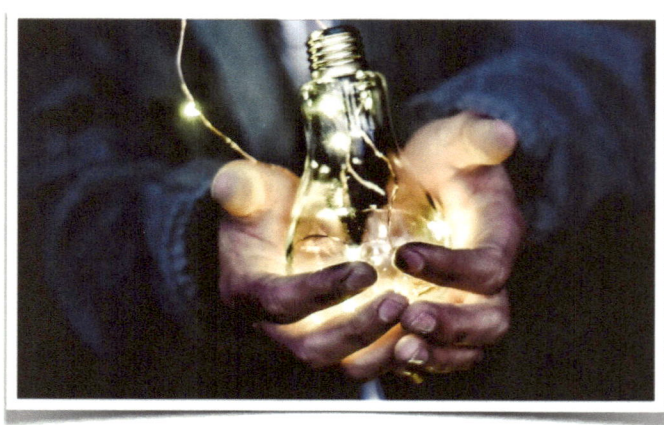

A few A few months ago I was training a client and we just hit it off really really fast. It wasn't because I was a therapist. It wasn't because I was bald. It wasn't because I told a bunch of funny jokes. It was because we had something in common. She was a Bible believing Christian and so am I. Therefore, we just clicked. It is not that we talked about the Bible frequently or for a long period time but we knew that we were like minded.

Can two walk together, except they be agreed? Amos 3:3

One sure fire way to get someone to agree with you is to find something that you both have in common. That is right. This may make commonsense, but common sense isn't always common practice. You want to be likable. I did not say you want them to like you. I said you want to be likable. This means that you simply want your client to know that you and them share a common interest. This will take some extra work on your part, but remember you are not seeking to be average, you are seeking to be extraordinary.

So, this is what I want you to do. I am sure you already have an idea of who this person is from the chart review. Now I want you to go a little bit deeper. What that means is that you are going to ask questions prior to asking them to do something for you. You are going to

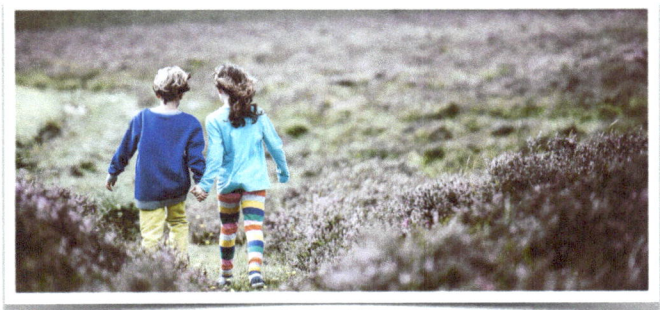

go on a scavenger hunt. You are searching for gold. You are searching for something that you can illuminate or bring to the surface that you and your client have in common. In his worldwide bestselling book titled Influence, Robert Cialdini, stated you need to bring something to the surface that you and the person you are attempting to influence have in common. He says that this will increase the likelihood of them saying yes to your ideas and requests. Isn't this exactly what we want to happen? We want to make it easy for our clients to say yes to whatever we ask them to do. We want them to say yes because we believe that what we request of them, will be in their best interest.

The reality is that most of us who are part of the human race have something in common with someone else. But, what happens is that we spend too much time illuminating the things that make us different. Our skin color makes us different, our sex makes us different, the clothes that we wear make us different, our accents make us different, and our social economical position make us different. All these things tend to separate us instead of bringing us closer. Our goal is for our clients to feel a pulling or attraction towards us. This attraction is created through something we have in common. It could be something as simple as they have on Nike tennis shoes and you just bought some Nike tennis shoes two days ago. Now you both are in a full-blown conversation about why you selected Nike tennis shoes. Now, even if they don't want to go with you or participate with you at this point, they are going to feel slightly uncomfortable saying no because, now you both are walking together in agreement. You have just made it easier for them to say yes, than to say no.

So now, this is another tool for you to put into your tool belt. You will no longer just begin making requests to people as if they are strangers. You are going to seek out something that you both have in common and make them into one of your friends. You are going to go above and beyond to find out more then the medical chart says about them. You are going to begin to see them as a person. You are going to begin to communicate with them as if they have a life outside of the current dysfunction. You are going to share with them something about you as you find out more information about them. This process will not be a part of your medical record and it will not increase your income. What this will do is cause you to be an awesome, amazing, and outstanding medical professional. That is because you have positioned yourself not just as someone that gets the job done, but someone who actually cares about the client as a person. Remember, your client is a person first and a patient second. If you attract the person, it becomes easier to heal the patient.

Chapter 3

MAKE THEIR GOAL YOUR PRIORITY

Where I work it is a big open gym. This is great for patient interaction with other patients but it is difficult for patient confidentiality. There are times when we have to whisper comments to patients knowing that there are other patients in the room listening. We of course want to make sure that all the information that we are sharing with the resident, as it relates to their medical condition, remains private. Now, this is the story about what happens almost all too often in the gym. It is time to perform gait training or transfer training and the individual says, they "don't want to, they're too tired, their in to much pain, or maybe we can just do this tomorrow." This happens pretty often to me as I'm sure it does to plenty of other clinicians. Now there are two ways that this can go. I can encourage them to stand up and walk anyway because it is the best thing for them to do, or I can remind them as to what their goals are and why they are here. Contrary to some clinicians belief, we are not the most important people in our clients lives. The most important person in our clients life is undoubtably themselves. They do not care what we want them to do, they care about what they want to do. The only reason why they are spending time with us today is that someone told them or they convinced themselves that we could get them what they wanted. What do they want? They don't want to suffer anymore, they want to walk, they want to return home, they want to get stronger, they want to restore some level of function that they thought was gone forever. My clients do not want to stand up and walk when they are tired and hurting just because I asked them to. They only want to do what they want to do.

Arouse in the other person an eager want. Dale Carnegie, How To Win Friends and Influence People

Dale Carnegie wants us to get a major point out of reading his breath taking book. He wants us to increase our "tendency to think always in terms of other people's point of view and to see things from their angle". You know to do this we must consistently remind ourselves and our clients what they want. We must have their goals on the forefront of our mind at all times. We must always work from the position of getting them what they want. Our clients don't want to feel like they're being forced into doing anything. They want to feel like they are being encouraged to do something that is in their best interest. Our clients also need to see a direct relationship between what we're asking them to do and what their goals are.

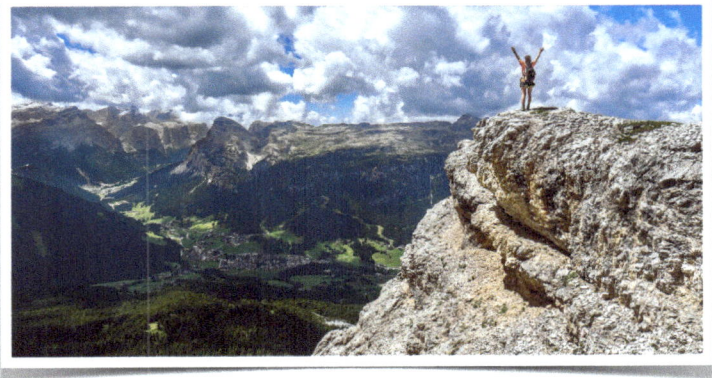

The only way that this relationship can remain clear is that we remind ourselves and our clients the importance of them reaching their goal.

So I'm sure the question has arisen in your mind. How do you arouse a patient or client to want something. How do you get them to really want whatever goal they have for themselves. As you know from experience a lot of people want things, but they do not want to put in the work to have those things. Mr. Carnegie suggest that we spend our time and conversations with our clients talking about what they want and how they could get it. Our entire conversations should be centered around them getting what they want. It doesn't matter if we are going to draw a patient's blood, or getting a patient dressed, or taking vital signs, or about to do a five minute ride on the bicycle. Everything that we are asking them to do should be centered around them getting what they want. If at any time there was any hindrance, or we see any type of non compliance, we should take stock of ourselves first and make sure that we are communicating in such a way that the client believes that we are working to get them what they want. Earlier in the book, How to Win Friends and Influence People, John Dewey, an American philosopher, was quoted as saying "the desire to be important" is the deepest urges in human nature. This goes right back to our original statement and concern. How do we encourage people to do what we want them to do? We make them feel important and remind them that we are giving them what they want.

The next time that you decide to go and see a patient or client make sure that you ask yourself, what does my client␣what and how can I communicate to them how they can have it. Over 90% of our communication with the patients should be the importance of their goals and how exactly we will help them achieve them.

Chapter 4

USE YOUR IMAGINATION

A few years ago there was a series of commercials that came out advertising headphones. The headphones were Beats by Dr. Dre. I really love these commercials because of the message more than because of the product. This particular commercial showed angry fans screaming and hollering at a professional athlete. They were yelling obscenities to him, the news reporters were stating how he should never play the game again, and every other thing that you could think of negative was being said. Then the athlete put on the headphones. Once the athlete put on the headphones all of the negative noise was silenced. He was reminded who he truly was. Nothing changed with his surroundings. The only thing that changed was the voice inside of his head. The title of the commercial was: "Hear What You Want." It was such a cool commercial because as you're watching it and see the aggravation the stress on his face based upon what everyone was saying to him, then see a small smile by the end of the commercial. What is so cool and exciting about this to us as clinicians, is that no matter what our clients say to us, we have the ability to imagine whatever we want. As you may know the brain does three things very very well. The brain deletes, distorts, and generalizes all the information that is given to us. It is up to us to use our imagination and filter out all the noise, so not only can we perform at a high level, but also not get distracted by all the negative noise that maybe coming from clients.

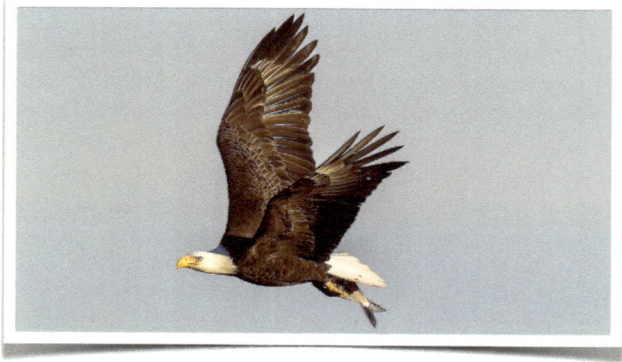

The man who has no imagination, has no wings. Muhammad Ali

In what way does this quote speak to you? Let me say this, it inspires me to think. As a clinician I am in a position to influence someone else to fly. I don't mean to walk, but I mean to fly. What it simply means is this, a client comes into your area of influence, you can causes them to feel bad, good, great or phenomenal. The way that you influence them to feel has nothing to do with what they say to you. It had everything to do with your interpretation of what they say to you, the meaning that you give the comments, and the use of your imagination. So let's stop for a second and not think about the likely or the expected performance of our clients based upon the medical records. Let's use imagination and if anything was possible,; how would our clients respond to us and how will they perform today. Let's push ourselves closer to the edge of what's possible as opposed to staying close to the shore where only average is expected.

Imagination is more important than knowledge. Albert Einstein

Did you see who said that? Albert Einstein himself said that imagination is more important than knowledge. When we approach our clients in Vegas situation we have all the knowledge that we need in order to provide excellent care. So what prevents us from providing excellent care all the time? It is our imagination. Our imagination causes us to think that they will not perform well, they will not want to do what we are asking them to do, and that the result of her inaction may be unfavorable. This is a grand miss use of our imagination. We are to use our imagination constructively in order to create the phenomenal experience that we want our clients to have. What does and interaction of high engagement look like to you? You must figure out what that is in your imagination first, if you are going to create it. Never go into a situation with the client without high expectations. And those high expectations begin in your imagination.

If you think you can do anything or if you think you can't do a thing you're right. Henry Ford

Now where does this thinking that we can or we can't start? It all stars in our imagination. As we walk into the room to see a patient our imagination has already decided what is going to happen. If we imagined that this is going to be a tough or negative interaction we are going to hold our bodies a certain way, our tone of voice is going to sound a certain way, and even the expression on her face will be different. So just as a fun little experiment, I want you to spend time imagining the most excellent interaction with each and everyone of your clients or patients before you see them. If you are seeing them for just being a couple seconds before you walk in the room or before you around the corner, imagine a successful interaction between him and excitement that this interaction is going to entail. I want you to bring the excitement in the room. I want you to bring the joy, the comfort, the likability, and the enthusiastic imagination of a high level of engagement. Remember, The situation does not control your imagination; the meaning you give to the situation controls by your imagination. Make a decision to give a positive meaning to every situation even before it begins.

Chapter 5

EXPECT THE RESULTS YOU WANT

Welcome to the final chapter of this short book. I hope that you have learned something and have enjoyed the journey. Now we continue on to the last aspect of client engagement.

I have a few children of my own and I have the awesome responsibility to care for them and to homeschool them (with about 99.9% of Homeschooling done by my wife). Everyone knows they are required to take exams and that always creates an interesting emotional response. There have been a few times when before they even saw any questions on the exam they expected not to do well. The only way that I can wrap my head around this is that, maybe they didn't prepare well. But, that's not the case. It is not that they haven't studied, or haven't reviewed the information. The fact of the matter is they just don't expect to do well. They have to exercise their imagination so that they can see themselves doing well. Therefore, it has been my focus for a number of years, to teach them how to expect to win.

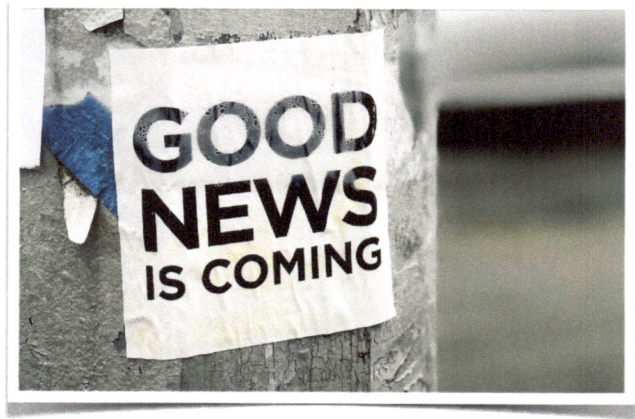

High expectations are the key to everything. Sam Walton

Oh yes, Sam Walton said a mouthful. High expectations! Do you have high expectations? This quote in my opinion is not talking about the high expectations I am to have a my children or the high expectations that you are to have of your patients. A lot of times, we have high expectations for other people and therefore we get disappointed. But, what about the expectations we have of ourselves. In this chapter I want to encourage and inspire you to raise your level of expectation of yourself. I want you to expect to create a trusting environment with each and everyone of your clients. I want you to expect to focus on what's most important with each and everyone of your clients. I want you to expect you to arouse enthusiasm in each and everyone of your clients and bring out the best in them. I want you to expect yourself to go the extra mile and find something that you have in common with your client. I want you to have high expectations for every aspect of your professional career. You may never be able to control the atmosphere that you're working in but you can control your interpretation of the atmosphere. You are going to have clients that are unruly and some that just don't progress the way that you thought that they should. In spite of all of that I want you to challenge yourself to remain in a state of high expectation of engaging action on your part.

Now is the time for you to put a stake in the ground. For you to take a stand. For you to demand more of yourself than you ever have before. This is the time for you to see something in yourself that you have never seen before. This is your time to become the champion that you always wanted to be. Now is the time for you to step out from the crowd of average and set yourself up to be the very best version of yourself possible. It is time for you to live at the highest level! But how do you live at the highest level possible and expect more of yourself?

I think the ability of the average man could be doubled if it were demanded... Will Durant

Wow! Did you just read that, the way that I read it? The way that you live at the highest level possible is to place higher demands on your self. And, that is what this book has been all about. You have learned things that will cause you to demand more of yourself. You just can't go to a client or patient just any kind of way anymore. Now you go with intention each and every encounter. With each and every encounter you are expecting a positive result. A positive or great results doesn't mean that it's going to feel good. What it means is that there will be progress. The benefits come from you working harder than you've ever worked before, to increase the level of client engagement. The more attention that you give, the person, the level of client engagement will increase. You will begin to see results. It may not happen the first time you do it, but all hard work yields a profit.

As I conclude, I want to encourage you just one more time. As a medical professional you have been entrusted with a great responsibility. Millions and millions of people are suffering. The people that are suffering need someone that not only is intelligent but someone that also has a heart. A heart that genuinely cares for the person on the other side of the pain. My final series of questions to you are as follows: Are you the one? Are you the one that will prioritize the person and not your scheduled agenda? Are you the one that will step outside of your comfort zone or outside of the way you always do things, as to attempt a different way? Some people will say that they tried it and it didn't work. Some people say that it's too hard. Some people say that is not worth the effort to even try. But, what will you say? Make your decision right now to do it or not to do it. The choice is yours to make.

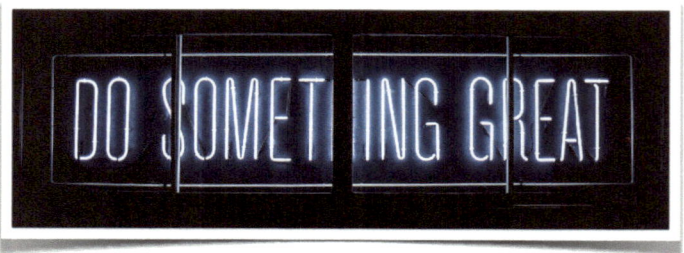

There is no try. There is either do or do not! Yoda

CHOOSE TO BE average or choose to be EXTRAORDINARY!

Your friend

Lynn Pierre

REFERENCES

Chapter 1:

The Treasury of Quotes by Jim Rohn

Chapter 2:

Influence: The Psychology of Persuasion by Robert Cialdini

How to Win Friends and Influence People by Dale Carnegie

Holy Bible: KJV

Chapter 3:

How to Win Friends and Influence People by Dale Carnegie

Chapter 4:

NLP: The Essential Guide by NLP Comprehensive and Tom Dotz

Chapter 5:

One Decision Separates The Wealthy from the Non-Wealthy (blog) by Benjamin P. Hardy

RECOMMENDED READING:

How to Win Friends and Influence People by Dale Carnegie

High Performance Habits by Brendon Burchard

The 7 Day Mental Diet by Emmet Fox

Drive: The Surprising Truth About What Motivates Us by Daniel H. Pink

Sell or be Sold: How to Get Your Way in Business and in Life by Grant Cardone

100 Ways to Motivate Yourself: Change Your Life Forever by Steve Chandler

Holy Bible

The Power of Habit: Why We Do What We Do in Life and Business by Charles Duhigg

ABOUT MEDICAL EMPOWERMENT INSTITUTE

Our primary objectives are to educate (CEUs), provide a great experience, and empower medical professionals to do what they do at the highest level possible. We serve individual clinicians as well as business and corporations. Our emphasis is on the following:

- Positive and Empowering Thoughts
- Actions of Enthusiasm
- High Levels of Engagement
- Demanding Growth and Progression
- Intentional Listening
- Creating and Walking in a Vision
- Developing Oneself
- Focus and Emotional Control

We believe that as the individual clinician invest in him/herself they will be in a better position to give more of themselves to their clients, their craft, and their community. All of this works together to raise the standard of practice in each medical discipline.

We provide the following:

- Live Educational Events
- On-Site Events
- Department and Individual Coaching

For more information, to join use at our next event, or to schedule an event at your location, please visit www.medpowerinstitute.com or email us at info@medpowerinstitute.com.

OUR TRUSTED PARTNERS

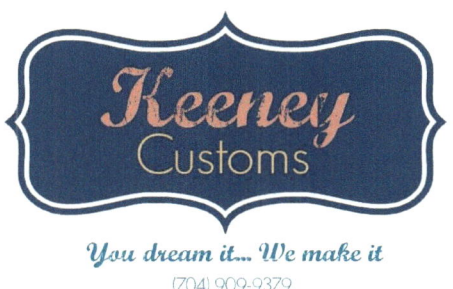

We are a family business with a passion for creating custom designs of all kinds. Our goal is to create exceptional designs using good quality materials to unleash your creative vision. From t-shirts to tumblers, home decor & gifts..let us customize it for you.

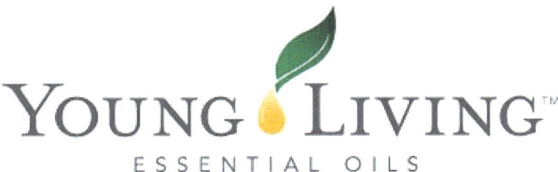

Young Living is a universally known, household name that is revered and respected for the countless benefits it brings to humanity. Propelled by the world's purest essential oils and oil-infused products, along with our passionate commitment to empowering individuals to whole-life wellness, we champion the modern essential oil movement. A global, purpose-driven wellness revolution is underway, and Young Living leads the charge.

Member # 14934251

www.ingramcontent.com/pod-product-compliance
Lightning Source LLC
Chambersburg PA
CBHW040344220526
45473CB00009B/2780